Brain
Surgery
And
Recovery
From
A
Patient's
Point of
View

Brain
Surgery
And
Recovery
From
A
Patient's
Point of
View

Delores Beecham

Library of Congress Control Number:		1-234791651
ISBN:	Hardback	978-1-4415-8623-0
	Softcover	978-1-4415-7219-6

This book was printed in the United States of America.

To order additional copies of this book, contact:
Xlibris Corporation
1-888-795-4274
www.Xlibris.com
Orders@Xlibris.com
68410

TABLE OF CONTENTS

(An autobiography of the events leading to including and after both brain surgeries)

INTRODUCTION

My guess is you selected this book because someone you know has had brain surgery, is about to undergo brain surgery, or you are about to undergo brain surgery. I think it is wise of you to learn more about brain surgery. In this book, I will tell you my story and hope you will do the right thing. I wrote this book so you and your loved ones can understand fully what you are up against. I believe I am qualified because I have gone through two brain surgeries within seven months. I learned a great deal and some of it might help you and your loved ones get through this as effortless and painless as possible. I won't tell you it's easy. It's not. I'd be dishonest if I did. What you do need to consider is putting your trust in God and believing everything is going to be fine. A positive attitude and prayer are the best things you and your loved ones can do for one another. If a book such as this had been available and I knew about it, I would have been grateful. I wouldn't have been so frightened. After you have been diagnosed with a brain tumor, don't put off the inevitable. The sooner you have this taken care of, the better you will feel. The tumor isn't going away, it will only get worse. Medication can only do so much. The growth has to be removed so you can get on with your life or lives. In future chapters, I will disclose some things you should do and not do that will make your recovery easier.

DEDICATION

This book is dedicated to my fiancé Charles with love. Charles was such an inspiration before during and after both brain surgeries. I'm sure had it not been for him and his loyal support, I would not be around today to help other brain tumor patients, their families and loved ones get through this very delicate time in their lives. With God's help I might be able to save some lives, that is my desire.

ACKNOWLEDGEMENTS

First, I'd like to say thank you to God. Paula, my eldest daughter, you were there in my time of need. Thank you for your loyalty. You shall be rewarded. Teresa, my youngest daughter, I'm sure you handled the situation to the best of your ability. Tyrone, my son, may God Bless you and keep you. To my parents, H. Matthew Beecham and Esther M. Beecham. Thank you for your special prayers. To my long time friend who has been in my life for decades I like to say thank you, Myra for your wisdom and understanding. To all my friends and relatives too numerous to name. Thank you. I love you. To the staff of surgeons, doctors, technicians and nurses at the Memorial Hospital of Long Beach, CA. I thank you for your knowledge and special skills.

THE BRAIN

Without attempting to practice medicine, let me tell you a few things about the human brain. The brain is a very small yet complex part of your nervous system housed within your skull. The brain is the motor of your being. The brain controls your emotion and send signals throughout your body. The brain determines whether or not something is hot or cold, sharp or dull. It controls love, hate, sadness or gladness. Without your brain you would be like the scarecrow in the Wizard of Oz. If I have relayed the message intended, I hope you will take care of your health, including your brain.

TUMORS

If you have been diagnosed as having a brain tumor, I know you have been through several test and have a lot of questions to ask your doctor. Ask away. That's why they are there. Get several opinions if you desire, because I'm sure you hope the first one is incorrect. If you have not seen a doctor and you're wondering if you have a brain tumor because you have some of the symptom's you heard about, forget it, see your doctor and let him/her tell you what you need to know. A tumor does not have to be malignant. A tumor is a growth, so is a hang nail as told to me by my doctor. With today's advanced technologies and surgical procedures and the frequency the surgery is being performed, the surgery could almost be classified as minor (almost).

HEADACHES

Not all headaches are brain tumors. Some headaches are caused by anxiety, stress, allergies, poor vision, scents, the elements and numerous other things in this life. What I'm suggesting to you as the patient is: if you're suddenly experiencing long painful and unusual headaches don't hesitate to see your physician immediately and insist on something more than medication. You know your body better than anyone else when it comes to pains, aches and unusual behavioral patterns. A very early diagnosis can save you and your family much anguish. An early detection could save your life.

MEDICATION

You will probably be prescribed medications, at least one. The directions will be on the container or vile follow the directions precisely. Most medications are to be taken three times daily. Try and arrange these medications around meals. Most medications have side effects. Ask your doctor to explain what they are although the information may be found on the pamphlet that accompanies your medications (e.g. some make you gain weight, some cause you to have a dry mouth) to name a few, with the weight gain, cut back on your food intake. To prevent ulcers, it helps to never take medication on an empty stomach. If you're experiencing a dry mouth, drink plenty of fluids preferably water, suck on a sugarless mint or chew gum. If you have any problems such as dizziness, rashes, insomnia or upset stomach, give your doctor's office a call. The doctor might have to reduce your dosage or prescribe another medication. There are several medications the doctor might make available to you. If at any time you change doctors, carry a list of your medications to your new doctor. Make sure you advise the doctor of the medications that you are allergic to. As a new patient, you will have forms to fill out depending on your condition. You might be wise to take a close friend or family member with you.

VEINS

If you have been told by a doctor or technician your veins are not good and they have a hard time drawing blood or inserting an IV, do a lot of hand exercises. The particular exercise I recommend is lifting hand weights. I think you can do this while recuperating in bed, or just watching television. The size of the weights depends on your size. I suggest the women use the smaller weights. But get weights that will be a little strenuous so you will notice the pull. The five pound weights should do nicely. After all, you are trying to get your veins back to normal not compete in a body building contest. The body builders know more about weights than I can tell them. The same rule, in my estimation would apply. Get weights you know will be a little strenuous. My anesthesiologist gave me this advice when he noticed the bruises on my hands and arms, in which the technicians and nurses had made while trying to find my veins. For whatever reason, I believe in my heart so many of them knew less about what they were doing than others. When I went home I got out my dumbbells and proceeded to use them. My weights are five pounds. I did these exercises while still in bed recuperating. I would take the weights and move my hand one at a time back and forth, side to side being very careful. After I finished one hand I would do the other. I would do these exercises twice daily until I became stronger. I can attest to these weights doing exactly what my doctor said they would do. Now that I know about the weights, hopefully they will not have any difficulty finding good veins again.

THE WALK IN PATIENT

Make sure you carry your insurance carrier information with your phone numbers of friends, relatives, significant others etc., if you wear glasses or contacts, wear or carry them because you will be filling out new patient information. Your family can take your belongings home and return them to you at a later time. The hospital is not responsible for your valuables. Here are a few things to pack in an overnight bag to be brought to you later comb, brush, robe, slippers, toothpaste, toothbrush and soap if you prefer your own. The hospital furnishes soap, deodorant and shampoo. You might be there long enough to wash your hair if it was not shaven. A book to read would be nice, head covering to wear home and some change for newspaper and mints. I advise no more than three dollars at a time. Someone can bring more as your time in the hospital increases. I never mentioned a gown or pajamas because the hospital gown is more convenient and suitable for all the doctors, nurses and technicians that want to examine and do test on you.

THE UNCONSCIOUS TO
SEMI-CONSCIOUS PATIENT

If the patient has been carried to the hospital from an accident scene and you are the first person to be notified, try to compose yourself so you will be able to answer pertinent questions that are asked of you about the patient. If you are not a relative, get in touch with a relative as soon as you can. Most hospitals don't recognize friends when making decisions about impending surgery. Most people carry some type of identification in their wallet or purse. Some of this information might be insurance related that may be used to take care of the much needed emergency treatment at that time. If the patient has dentures, glasses or contact lenses, take special care and handling of these items. The clothing the patient was wearing might have to be cut off so be prepared. More clothing may be brought back for the trip home. Pack an overnight bag to be brought to the hospital.

THE SURGERY DAY

Whether you spend the night before surgery at home or in the hospital, after midnight you can't take anything by mouth. This is very important! You can't even chew gum. If you are taking medications, ask your doctor beforehand which ones you are allowed to take. Very early in the morning, usually your surgery day begins. The nurses will get you prepared for surgery by administering medication, giving you a change of clothing, surgery clothes, and a cap to be placed on your head. You are asked to help the nurses or technicians move yourself from the bed to the gurney and you are wheeled to the operating room which is the surgery floor. There you will be placed in a room call the holding room. One special visitor can stay with you there. You will have your vitals taken, surgical stockings will be placed on your legs (depending on your doctor). A warm blanket can be placed on you if you so desire. Knowing you are going to surgery automatically gives you the shakes and makes you cold. You will be asked many questions about your current medications and allergic reactions to them. This is where you are introduced to your anesthesiologist and he or she asks more questions and inserts IV's into your arms. About this time you are wheeled into the operating room. You don't even know if the medication has begun to work. Several hours have passed, but to you it seems as if it were only a few minutes. Later your surgery is over and you are in the recovery room. You will be given a lot of attention. You will go in and out of consciousness. You will feel hands all over you. You are being checked from head to toe. You don't even have to worry about going to the bathroom. All of that is being taken care of for you. You'll probably have a catheter inserted. This room will be your home for a few days. When you are better, you will be placed in a semi-private to private room. Here your head will be elevated slightly and may be on oxygen. Visiting hours are different than on the regular floor. After you're better, you might be asked to squeeze the nurse's hands, move your feet and blow into a bottle. You might also be asked a lot of questions (e.g. where are you? what day is it? what is your address? what is your name?) just to mention a few. These questions are being asked of you to see how well your surgery went. All your answers and all you do, is being written down so your doctor can see how you are progressing.

THE LONG WAIT FOR FRIENDS

AND RELATIVES OF THE PATIENT

Be sure to wear something comfortable because your wait is going to be very long and tiring. A book, magazine, games or knitting might be helpful. If you like listening to the radio, or if you have an ipod, bring it along. Some hospitals have televisions in the waiting rooms. The channel might not be set on your favorite channel. Therefore, you might not appreciate it. Bring company along if possible. Someone to talk to would be advantageous, time would pass faster. Surgery can take anywhere between three and six hours possibly more depending on the procedure being done. If you live relatively close, you could go home and return later. I would not advise it though. I know you're not supposed to think negatively, but anything could happen and you would be very saddened if you were not there when the doctor came to tell you the news. The doctor will let you know approximately how long the surgery is going to take. After the doctor has done the surgery and told you of the patient's condition, you can then go home if you choose. The patient will be recovering and not aware you're there for several hours. You might want to have a few telephone numbers handy. Some relatives that couldn't make it might want to know the results before too long. You can give them the results of the surgery as the doctor gave them to you. Never, I mean never wait for a surgery patient alone.

TO THE FAMILY AND FRIENDS
OF A BRAIN SURGERY PATIENT

A brain surgery patient might be a little confused at times. Behavioral patterns may be altered somewhat. Try to be understanding. The fact that the patient has gone through brain surgery is depressing enough. Moods suddenly change for no apparent reason. Be kind, say a few words of encouragement. Let the patient know everything is going to be fine. If you can't think of anything to say, a hug, a pat on the shoulder or back, a kiss or handshake would be welcomed. Some of these things might seem insignificant to a well person, but to a brain surgery patient, these things can mean a lot. Young children should not be allowed to see the patient too soon after surgery. I know the hospital has rules, but rules always get broken. The sight of some brain surgery patients to a young child is not good. The head has been shaven and the head might be completely bandaged depending on the surgery and doctor. The eyes are more than likely dark and swollen. A patient usually is not able to walk or talk. If they talk at all, the phrases may be slurred. Sometimes the arms, hands and feet are affected. For instance, a young child was happily playing with his/her parent two days before surgery. The parent appeared normal, now the child sees his/her parent lying here in this altered condition. This will leave a definite effect on the child. The child might have emotional problems later. The child could have bad dreams.

As adults, it is our place to comfort our children the best of our ability (or the best we know how). When visiting a patient, be considerate. Don't overstay your welcome, or visit. The patient is unable to tell you they are tired. Use some discretion. As a patient, you're constantly being visited by doctors, nurses, laboratory technicians, food service workers, priests and other visitors all asking questions. I'd like to say to you, all that attention really makes a patient tired. If at all possible, make sure only two people visit at one time. When more than two people visit they all sometimes talk at once. It gets to be tiring. One nice thing you can do for a patient is bring a small tape player or ipod with some of their favorite music for them to listen to. Some of this music reminds them of being home and having better days. If you have an answering machine, perhaps some of the messages of familiar voices will be helpful. The radio music in the hospital is just that, hospital music. The television is a joke after brain surgery. The television is the last thing you want to see. Also, sometimes patients have to share a television. While visiting the patient, if you can be of assistance to them help with hand exercises, fluff a pillow get an extra blanket and assist them in walking if allowed. If a patient can get in a wheelchair, wheel them to the sun room or outside if the weather permits. Comb or brush their hair, apply lotion, do whatever you can to make your visit count.

YOUR DISCHARGE

FROM THE HOSPITAL

Today is your discharge day and I'm sure you're excited. The doctor told you several days ago that today you could go home. This morning you woke up especially early getting your personal things together and primping a little more than before. Your discharge papers must be signed by your doctor first. Perhaps this has already been done. Lists of medications have to be listed or prescriptions made out. You must have someone pick you up. I'm sure all this has been pre-arranged by your family. A wheelchair will be brought to your room to escort you to your vehicle. Be sure to take everything you paid for, if you want them such as pitchers, cups, tissues, wash basin, urinal, egg crate, mattress pad, soap etc.

AFTER YOU'RE HOME

You are home. Remember, you are still a sick person and you will have to take the best care of yourself you know how. Remember to keep your head elevated slightly. This is still important. Do a lot of deep breathing exercises to keep the lungs strong and prevent pneumonia. Inhale and exhale through your mouth as you would for your doctor when taking a physical. These exercises also help keep the lungs fluid free. Cough when you can. You might cough up mucous and phlegm which will only help you to a speedier recovery. Don't get despondent. Getting despondent can only work against your recovery. With any surgery, the patient has to give their surgery time to heal and a reasonable amount of time to feel like their old self again. Don't expect too much too soon and don't give up. I heard somewhere once "quitting is bad for your health". I thought that was a very appropriate saying. As for your scar, ask your doctor when and what he/she would suggest you use. I used cocoa butter and vitamin E oil alternately. I had very good results. If you feel something else would work better for you, use it. My scar healed nicely, my hair grew back and is undetectable that brain surgery was ever performed. I was satisfied with the results, and I have promising expectations that the second scar will heal with equal success.

MY OWN TRUE STORY

I first went to my family doctor on June 1, 1987 because I was having severe headaches. I was suspicious because I never had headaches such as those. I was out of town with my eldest daughter Paula, when the first headache occurred. In the middle of the morning, I was awakened by a very sharp pain in my head. I took two aspirin but the pain continued as if I had only taken a drink of water. I was frightened but I didn't disturb Paula because we didn't know where a doctor was in this strange town, plus I also didn't want to panic her as well as myself. After two hours or so, I dosed off to sleep; it wasn't a good sleep nevertheless. In the morning when Paula was up, I described this pain to her. I said to her "I have never had a stroke, nor do I know what a stroke feels like, but I thought early this morning I was about to experience what one felt like from the pain in my head". She said, "How do you feel now?" I replied, better. That day we went to Las Vegas. I drove even though I still had the headaches. I thought if I got out of town and drove the pain would lessen. I was wrong. We stayed about two hours then we went back to where we were staying. It was about one and half hours away from Las Vegas.

I'll never forget that day. It was Memorial Day 1987. The next day we headed home. I drove. I thought I could ease the pain by driving. I'll always remember this pain as long as I live. This was the most excruciating pain in my life. I'm a lady who has given birth three times and had teeth drilled and filled without Novocain and much more. We arrived home on June 1, 1987. The first person I wanted to see was my doctor. Charles couldn't help me now. I called and made an appointment with my family physician that Monday morning since I was unable to go to work. The doctor examined me and gave me medication and took me off work for four days. I could hardly lift my head off the pillow. The fifth day I reported to work, the medication the doctor had prescribed wasn't working, my headache got worse. Two weeks later, I reported back to my doctor and told him the medication wasn't working. I was still experiencing pain in my head. My doctor ordered x-rays for sinus but those x-rays were normal. The doctor changed my medication. Four days later, I was in my doctor's office again. The doctor said he was ruling out brain tumor because I had been his patient for three years and I didn't have a history of headaches. A week later I decided to see my Ear, Nose and Throat doctor. I was told by him, since I had nose surgery in 1985, it was possible that was causing my headaches. I accepted this diagnosis because I needed an answer. He then prescribed nose spray. A month or so passed. I was on medication from two doctors so the headaches subsided somewhat. I continued to have headaches, but not nearly as severe. Two and a half months passed. On my way home from after working a 10 hour shift, I was involved in a small accident. I hit the back of another car. The lady I hit was a fellow employee. Neither she nor I were injured. We looked at the vehicles, exchanged information and decided the damage was nil. We agreed, let's try to make it home safely after this and smiled. I stopped in a nearby department store to make several purchases because Charles and I were going out of town that weekend. When I reached a telephone, I called Charles and made him aware of the small accident I was just involved in. I proceeded to tell him about the accident and he said to me "what's wrong" I said nothing except the accident. I suppose I was a little shaken up. Charles replied "you're more than a little shaken up". You sound like someone else. Do you want me to come take you home he said? I insisted I was fine besides Charles was at work for the day. I told him I would call when I arrived home. This was the last day to weigh in at weight watchers. I'm a life time member and have to weigh in once a month. My weight was fine. On my way home from weight watchers before I reached home, I was involved in a second accident. After I hit this vehicle, I guess I must have hit my mouth on the steering wheel. A man came running to my vehicle which was a truck, asking me if I were okay. I said "yes". He asked because I was bleeding from my mouth and I had no idea. My vehicle was stalled in the flow of traffic. I recall someone asking me if I could steer, I couldn't. They pushed and steered my vehicle out of traffic. I remember asking the lady I hit to call Charles but there were no telephones nearby, so she couldn't. Shortly a highway patrolman came and asked me a lot of questions I couldn't answer. He interrogated the mess out of me. I again asked if he would call Charles. He said his unit wasn't equipped to call any place except the station. After asking me questions I couldn't answer, he asked me if I wanted him to get in touch with the paramedics, I replied "No". The officer drove me to my home. I explained to him I have vertigo (motion sickness) and can't ride in the back seat. I recall throwing up in the unit. This, I thought was good. Children were outside playing and the officer asked them if any of them knew me and they replied "Yes". At this time my neighbor and her husband Linda and Johnny, came to my rescue. I asked them to call Charles at work. I guess they did. After that I didn't remember a thing. Charles was able to leave work in the company truck. He came home and carried me to the hospital emergency room where the doctors had to revive me because I had flat lined. The doctors asked Charles to leave, he did and returned the truck to work and clocked out. Charles got in his car and came back to the hospital to check on me. He spoke with the doctor and they told him they had moved me to the Intensive Care Unit of the hospital. He left and came back first thing the next morning to check on me. I don't remember any of this and the doctors said I probably wouldn't. What Charles, Paula and my cousin, Lucious have told me about the ordeal, I'm thankful I will never remember. Although, I do remember that my chest was sore as if someone had been jumping on it. After all the life saving maneuvers and what have you, I was released from the hospital after three days. I was having problems remembering. I had a brain concussion and there was brain damage. The brain tumor was diagnosed then. Two weeks later, I went for extensive brain test. The test the doctors recommended are called MRI and CT Scans. I was glad they weren't painful. I didn't know what to expect. I was placed in the cylinder and they strapped my head down. This wasn't painful. It was only a reminder to keep my head still. Dye was injected into my veins to shade the area they were observing. It was a piece of cake so to speak. When I went to the doctor, he told me the results of the test. Paula and Charles were there for support. I'm glad. I needed their support. The test disclosed I needed surgery and my doctors suggested I have it immediately. The next day the surgery was scheduled for nine days later. I didn't get a second opinion because I had already heard that Long Beach Memorial Hospital was the best hospital and the Neurologist local surgeon was also the best surgeon in the business. The hospital was excellent. When the president and their wives go to a hospital in California for treatment and procedures etc., this is the hospital they frequent. I received a citation through the mail from the municipal court regarding the accident I had caused due to my condition. The cost was $85.00. The date to appear was two weeks after my scheduled discharge from the hospital. The day before the surgery, I went to what is called Community Nursing. This is where you get all the test you will need for surgery; Chest X-Rays, Urinalysis, Blood work and everything your doctor requires. I did a lot of crying; I would wake up in the middle of the night and wished I could wake up from this bad dream. Most of my life I had been a healthy person. I wondered how this could be happening to me. I spent the last night before surgery at home so I would be comfortable in my own bed. I reported to the hospital at 6:00 a.m. the next morning. I had some final papers to sign before surgery. I had been approved for surgery by my insurance carrier, but right then, hospital didn't have the authorization. I had to sign papers stating that if the insurance carrier didn't pay, I would. I thought of canceling the surgery because I know I couldn't afford to pay. Charles said to me "It has been approved, don't worry" I did worry! After I had my name band attached, I was taken to another department where I undressed and they proceeded to prepare me further for surgery. All clothing and personals were taken off and had been taken home by Charles. I was given a bed where I was to wait for the anesthesiologist to sedate me. Charles waited there holding my hand and talking to me until I didn't remember anymore. After surgery the first thing I asked was "Did the insurance pay?" Charles said "Yes" don't worry. This time I didn't worry. Before, how could I not worry thinking I might have a seventeen thousand dollar hospital bill to pay. I was taken to intensive care where I remained for two and a half days being very closely monitored by my own private nurses. I was on oxygen, a heart monitor and an automatic blood pressure cuff. I recall going in and out of consciousness from the anesthesia. My throat was sore also from the anesthesia. I wanted ice cubes and damp towels on my mouth. I felt very dry. Paula was there constantly. I think the nurses wish they could have gotten rid of her. I really appreciated her being there. I said to her "I love you and I'm glad you are here" but where's Charles? Paula said its' okay, she understood. She said Charles had been there most of the morning and he left and went to work because he worked the night shift. The next time I awakened I saw him standing over me. I was conscious a very short time. I just hope anyone going through this have themselves a Charles or facsimile. On the night of the second day, I was moved to my room. Some tubes were removed. On the third day, my doctors visited me and encouraged me to do some walking. I was as weak as water. I walked to the bathroom with assistance. That was as far as I could go the first time out of bed. Each day I became stronger and stronger until I was able to walk without assistance. On the sixth day, I was released. The date was, October 1, 1987. I'll always remember that day. That was the day of the Whittier, CA earthquake. I was frightened, but why should I have been frightened what better place could I have been in? The building swayed back and forth. I just wanted to go home. Charles picked me up later and brought me home. I was glad to be home. At home everything was conveniently placed for me. A cooler was placed by my bedside filled with bottles of juices, fruit, water and ice. Breakfast was brought to my bedside every morning anything and everything I wanted. If we were out of it and I wanted it, Charles would go to the store and purchase it for me. I was still having problems; each time I moved too briskly I would experience pain in my head. I had to remember to take it easy. One week after I was home, my insurance representative came to my home and presented me with a check for the loss of my vehicle. Two weeks after I was discharged, I had to appear in court. I pleaded not guilty. The judge gave me a hearing date for three weeks later. One month after surgery, I, Paula and Charles went to Arizona where I had a vacation home. The trip lasted two days. We drove. When we returned home, I had a scheduled appointment to see my surgeon. After examining me, he said everything was fine, but I couldn't return to work yet nor could I drive. The next night, I started getting headaches. I guess I panicked. I called both daughters and Charles at work. Paula called my medical doctor, he prescribed medication for pain. My son Tyrone brought it over. I was encouraged to be in his office the next morning. We were. My doctor scheduled me for more test that same afternoon that we were there. The results were good. No change had been observed since the last three months earlier "Thank God", I said. When my court date arrived, there were no witnesses, so the judge said my case was dismissed see the bailiff. The bailiff told me I would be getting $85.00 in the mail within the next two weeks. I was glad. Within the next couple of months or so, I was going back and forth to doctors. I went to a doctor who gave me a spinal tap. This wasn't so great. I had to rest my head or I would experience headaches. I did rest a couple of days. A week later, I elected to have eye surgery. I wanted to do this on my own. My eyes were tearing constantly. I wanted to put a stop to this if at all possible. I had the surgery and was released from the hospital the same day. This is called outpatient surgery. The insurance wanted it that way. The surgery had a three week recovery time. I still couldn't return to work. I felt I needed a break because I was getting stressed. My doctor authorized a couple weeks more. Paula and I returned to Arizona.

That was my get-a-way spot. I drove half the distance and Paula drove the remainder. Things went very well. Our trip was successful. By the time I thought I was ready to return to work, I received a telephone call from my insurance claims adjuster. The lady I hit and her attorney didn't want to settle for the amount of coverage I carried. I became very upset and my blood pressure was uncontrollable. I had to stay off work for a month for hypertension. By the time my blood pressure became normal, I started having headaches again. I went for more tests. The results were bad. The brain was abnormal and medication couldn't do anything for it. Yes, I was told I needed brain surgery again. Charles was with me and I just fell apart. I asked questions. I asked if the surgery could be postponed and if I had the surgery this time would I become a vegetable. The surgeon said if you don't have the surgery, you will become a vegetable. I just loved the way he put his words. I had no choice except have the second surgery. Nine days later I checked into the hospital. This time I made sure the hospital had the authorization from my insurance carrier before I went into surgery. With this surgery, I didn't want to tell anyone. I had to tell my father because he knew I was going in for the test and he wanted to know the results. I spared my mother the grief. My cousin Florence, in Wisconsin wanted to know because I didn't tell her about the first surgery. When I called to tell her, she broke down and cried and so did I, her reply was, I'm supposed to be here for you and look at me. I told her that's why I didn't tell you the first time. My daughters knew about the first surgery but I didn't want to trouble them with this second surgery. Teresa had just lost a baby through miscarriage and I didn't figure she needed anymore grief. Paula had recently started a new job and a foreign language class. She also, had a four year old son Michael. I didn't want to burst her bubble by telling her the bad news. My son was out of town in the navy. Charles, bless his heart was the only close one to me that knew about the second surgery. I know now that was a mistake. That was a load too large for him to have to carry alone. During the surgery, he had to wait alone. There was no one there for him to talk to and console with. He waited there the entire time alone. I believe the surgery took three and a half hours. When I came out of recovery, I felt a lot better because I didn't go under thinking about having to pay the hospital bill if the insurance didn't. I didn't have to stay in intensive care but one day this time. The surgery went quite well considering. I think because I had the first surgery only seven months earlier. I was eating alone the next day after surgery. I was walking with assistance the second day. I was walking alone the third day. Two days after I came home, Charles left on vacation, it couldn't be avoided. The reservation was made two months prior before I knew I needed the surgery. I was able to take care of myself. Downstairs was prepared so I wouldn't have to go up the stairs. I was able to go upstairs after the second day. I took care of myself for two weeks. I couldn't drive. I had to ask my daughters for help only three times while Charles was away. Charles was gone exactly two weeks and four days. Believe me, I was counting the days because I was very lonely in as much as I didn't tell anyone. I learned a lesson from that. I believe I was the happiest person in the world when Charles returned. I was glad to be able to talk to someone about the surgery. I didn't suffer any. I just wanted to be able to talk to someone about how I felt. When someone did call and ask how I felt, I replied "fine" and that was that. I didn't elaborate. In fact, I would change the subject quite hurriedly and talk about something else. The next day, Charles returned to work; you see he's a workaholic. Even so, I was really glad to have him home. I was able to call on him at night at his job to talk to him. Out of state this would have been inconvenient. Four days later, I had an appointment to see my surgeon. The prognosis was good and he said I could return to work in a week and a half. I wasn't ready for work because I was feeling I couldn't cope with people especially people I worked with quite closely. My doctor said "you'll have to try it in order to get on with your life". If you don't go to work and see if you can perform the way you should, this will be a question that will always be on your mind if you don't. I still had the tubes in my nose from the eye surgery. I made an appointment to have the tubes removed. The doctor gave me three weeks to see the outcome of the surgery. I returned the day before the three weeks were up and the surgery was not the success we had hoped for. I returned to work the next day which was on a Thursday so I didn't have such a long week the first week back to work in over eleven months. Work went smoothly. I transferred from my previous department to another to make things more adjustable. I now had a new lease on life, so to speak. I was surrounded by a lot of new faces. I am blessed and grateful that

God spared my life. I believe He had a purpose in this life for me. I choose to believe He spared my life so I could help others by writing this book. To Him I will be eternally grateful. I procrastinated for twenty-two years. In this year of our Lord and Savior 2009, I'm writing this book with the help of my daughter Teresa and future daughter-in-law Roberta. I thank God I have them in my life to help with my book.

www.ingramcontent.com/pod-product-compliance
Lightning Source LLC
Chambersburg PA
CBHW021937170526
45157CB00005B/2332